HEALTHY by *Design*
Weight Loss, God's Way

Christian Weight Loss
Plan and Bible Study

Cathy Morenzie

Guiding Light Publishing

First Edition: July 2008
Second Edition: January 2011
Third Edition: December 2013
Fourth Edition: April 2015

ISBN: 978-0-9938888-4-7

Published by Guiding Light Publishing
261 Oakwood Ave, York, ON, Canada, M63 2V3

Note: The information in this book is for educational purposes only and is not recommended as a means of diagnosing or treating illness. All situations concerning physical or mental health should be supervised by a health professional knowledgeable in treating that particular condition. Neither the author nor anyone affiliated with Healthy by Design dispenses medical advice nor do they prescribe any remedies or assume any responsibility for anyone who chooses to treat themselves.

Cover Photo by: **Martin Brown Photography**
Cover and interior design: **Preston Squire Publishing Services**

Kick-Start your Weight Loss Journey

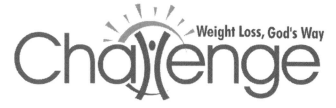

I'm inviting you to join our **FREE** *Weight Loss, God's Way Challenge* - a series of quick and easy videos, daily challenges and private discussions to help you to put your faith into action. This is my gift to you because if you're anything like me, you're probably read lots of books full of great strategies - without ever implementing what you've learned into your daily life. It's time to stop self-sabotaging and start reclaiming your health. Let's do it together in a loving, supportive, and prayerful atmosphere.

You will receive seven brief video messages from me, each with a humorous skit to powerfully show our weight loss mentality vs God's way. A daily challenge to get you to implement this book's principles into your life - now. Access to our powerful private discussion group. Plus our weekly newsletter full of practical and immediately useful Christian weight loss insights to keep you on track.

No commitment - you can unsubscribe at any time.

Valued at over $97, this gift is yours free!
Join now: www.weightlossgodswaybonus.com

Praying for your Success,

Cathy Morenzie

www.cathymorenzie.com

CONTENTS

FOREWARD

Like many of us, my journey of health, fitness and attempting to achieve and maintain a healthy weight, has been similar to a roller coaster ride. Plenty of ups, downs and unexpected curves which can leave your head (and heart!) spinning. There were times when I couldn't wait to step on the scale and times when, well, let's just say it fell into the 'not so pleasant' category.

Without a doubt, the greatest success that I have had on a long term, consistent basis was when working in partnership with Cathy Morenzie. Her God-given, cut to the chase, common sense approach to training, nutrition and balance has been an emotional and practical inspiration to me again and again. From writing down my goals, journaling my food intake, committing it all to God and keeping the long term goals in mind, I have developed into not only a goal setter, but a goal getter! You can add to that a six-time marathoner as well!

Praise the Lord, Cathy has decided to share her learning and experience that the Lord has blessed her with not only with her clients, but with us as well. In "Healthy by Design – Weight Loss, God's Way", she has compiled the wisdom gleaned from over twenty years of being a personal trainer and we stand to benefit immensely if we take it to heart.

Whatever your goal is (or goals are!), a number on a scale, that look of satisfaction in what you see in the mirror, fitting comfortably into a new or favorite outfit, honoring God with your eating habits and/or maybe even crossing a finish line, I want to encourage you: You can do it and there is assistance to be had! Using this book in your hands, you can see these dreams come to fruition and you will be blessed as a result.

On the faith and fitness journey,

Herbie Kuhn

Professional Sports Chaplain, Basketball Announcer & Impact Speaker

INTRODUCTION

The Problem

Do you have any idea how powerful you are? Have you ever thought about it? In Luke 10:19 Jesus says, *"I have given you authority to trample on snakes and scorpions and to overcome all the power of the enemy; nothing will harm you."* And that's just one of many scriptures that talks about the power we have in Christ.

So if we have all of this power and authority, why do we feel so powerless? How is it that we have been given the power and authority to cast out demons, yet we can't stop ourselves from eating a piece of chocolate? Why do we struggle with so many issues around our weight such as emotional eating, physical inactivity, self-control, guilt and feelings of low self-esteem?

A 2006 Purdue University study discovered that religious Americans were more likely to be overweight than their nonreligious peers. How can this be? Shouldn't we be the healthiest people on the planet because of the promises that God has given us? Where's the disconnect? The Purdue study indicated that many of the factors related to being overweight were associated with the increased social activities churchgoers participated in, such as after-church brunches and get-togethers. The fellowshipping with our fellow brothers and sisters is nice, but we need solutions to this health crisis. We don't need another church dinner, bake sale or barbecue.

The problem is analogous to having an air conditioner on a scorching hot day. We have been given an indispensable tool to help us but until we plug in the a/c, we will never receive the benefit and the power that exists at our disposal. Until we call on the Holy Spirit to be our help, as our instruction book tells us, we will never walk in the authority we have been given.

The Program

Healthy by Design: Weight Loss, God's Way is a 21 day workbook that will take you through the key principles of weight releasing based on biblical principles. To get the maximum benefit from the program you should carve out at least 20 minutes per day to complete the daily action steps. Take time throughout your day to reflect on the scripture. At the end of the day you should read it again and record your thoughts based on that topic.

The Daily Messages

The daily messages portray characters from the bible to teach us that our challenges are not unique; God understands them and wants to help us if we allow Him. They also teach us how faith plays an integral part in our lives and our victory.

The Daily Health Challenges

The daily health challenges are designed to make you think about where you are in your journey. They are designed to viscerally take you out of your habitual patterns and behaviors. To get the most out of the exercises be sure to put in the time to do them and reflect on the results. Be sure to have fun with them too.

The Daily Confession

The daily confessions provide an opportunity to speak God's word back to Him. They are all based on scripture and will help to change your though patterns about your health, your weight and your life in general.

An appendix is located at the back of the book where you can study additional scripture and mediate at your leisure on a particular area that might be a stronghold for you.

Continue through for 21 days straight - including weekends – if you skipped a day or had a day you didn't initially gain insight from, don't worry. Take as much time as you need on each chapter.

The Preparation

How are you feeling right now? You may be apprehensive, or excited, or perhaps having a fear of failing (again). In the course of this program you may go through a roller-coaster ride of emotions. I encourage you to keep a journal handy to write out any feelings that may come to the surface. Ask the Holy Spirit to reveal new truths and insights to you and to gently change you.

Throughout the workbook, avoid the tendency to judge yourself, your actions or your choices. There will be no right or wrong, no guilt or condemnation (*Romans 8:1*) - just notice what comes up for you and invite the Holy Spirit to make you present to your feelings; to show you the root of your stronghold(s) (*Psalm 139:23-24*) and to gird you for the journey.

You may choose to add the discipline of fasting. It is not a formal part of this program but if you are versed in fasting and feel confident that it will not be a distraction to you, then go ahead and add it in. Remember, fasting is not a weight loss tool but a means to help you draw closer to God so you can gain a better understanding of your weight challenges and banish them forever.

Avoid the urge to try to suddenly eat in a dramatically different way. Remember that there are no quick fixes to anything. Change is a process. You will learn that "trying" is rarely successful. Flesh can't change flesh but the Holy Spirit can help you if you will let Him. He is ready and available to you 24/7 if you call on Him to help you.

Are you familiar with the expression, "sow where you want to go"? It means that you should begin to do the action that you want to see manifest in your own life.

Begin to pray for other people also going through this process and know that they will be praying for you.

The Process

The goal of this program is to promote permanent change, through a series of small do-able incremental changes—baby steps.

This program will run for 21 consecutive days, but remember that this is only the beginning. You are on a life-long journey!

Each day you will read the weight loss principle, recite the daily confession and follow through on the daily action step. Remember, there are no quick fixes. You simply have to put in the time to allow growth and change to take place.

Please understand that this is not a book to teach you about exercises or foods that will help you lose weight. I'm willing to bet that you already know those answers. Instead you will learn the patterns, behaviors and mindsets that keep you stuck in same cycle of gaining and losing weight. Along with the ageless biblical principles to overcome those mindsets that have kept you in bondage.

The Principles

God has given us immutable laws and principles to govern our lives. These principles apply to everyone, every situation and every circumstance. Even if you do not practice them per se, you will still experience the consequences if you go against them. Use these principles in your weight releasing journey and other areas of your life to experience the victory, freedom and peace that God has already given you.

God wants to transform our lives little by little. Weight releasing is a process! - 2 Corinthians 3:18

There's nothing inspiring or motivating about the thought of slow and steady- especially when it comes to weight loss.

Though it may have taken us years to gain weight, we want to lose it fast. However, to be successful, we must understand that losing weight is a process. It will not happen overnight and we must gird ourselves to understand that the process will take a while. 2 Cor. 3:18 teaches us that God's glory comes in levels or stages when we partner with the Lord's spirit.

Though there are many instantaneous miracles that happen in the bible, we should understand that the qualities that God needs to develop in you to make your weight loss permanent will not happen miraculously. They need to be rehearsed and become engrained into your subconscious mind. As frustrating as it may seem, it will take some time but know that God has given you the capacity to be patient in the process once you submit the process to Him.

Understand that though the process may seem slow, the Word tells us that God is not slow in fulfilling his promises. (2 Peter 3:9) God will work in tandem with your obedience, so get ready to receive what He has for you – right away!

God wants us to partner with the Holy Spirit to live a victorious life. - John 14:15-25

In this scripture, Jesus tells his disciples that God will send the Holy Spirit, who will live with us, and be in us always. He will guide us, and be our advocate and helper. If you've tried to release weight on your own then you know that it can be a frustrating process often with more failures than successes. Now imagine letting go of all the anxiety and frustration; no longer living by letting the number on the scale determine the type of mood you will be in.

Imagine the confidence and peace you will feel at a social function. God's rich promises can all be yours when you allow the Holy Spirit to partner with you in this and every other stronghold in your life.

God has provided us with choices and He wants us to choose the best way. - Deuteronomy 30:19

Action/Consequences—from Adam and Eve to Revelations, God gives us the choice between right and wrong, blessings and curses. God created us with free will and would never impose His will on us. He lets us decide the choices we will make in life. Through our choices we learn wisdom and understanding.

Though it's not always obvious, many of the choices we make will bring blessings or curses. Choosing to sleep in, have an extra slice of cake or skip another workout are not curses in and of themselves, but they will weaken your disciple muscle which will eventually lead to poor health.

Conversely (and fortunately), taking the time to eat a proper breakfast, minimizing your intake of coffee, processed foods and sugar, and exercising regularly will not miraculously bring blessings to your life but will help you feel better, increase your energy and your mood, help you manage your weight and build your self-esteem which will have many long term blessings.

It may seem daunting right now but rest assured that God will teach you how to make good choices that will richly bless your life.

God wants to use our good health to glorify Him and to be an example to others. 1 Corinthians 6:19-20

God dwells in our physical bodies and calls it His temple. A temple is a sacred place of beauty and majesty. God took great pride and joy in creating us and He also want us to treat our bodies as the sacred temple He designed them to be.

We've all looked at other people and wondered how they could be Christians when they (insert vice here). Although God himself is not judging or condemning you, you probably know within yourself that you're not being as effective as you want to, because your weight is getting in the way.

You know that you would have more confidence, energy, stamina and effective witnessing when you are living at the level of health that God created you to live in.

The Purpose

Americans spend $40 billion a year on weight-loss programs and products. You probably have spent hundreds if not thousands yourself on products or programs promising you fast results.

You need a solution for how to release the weight without falling for sales gimmicks and unhealthy diets. What if I told you that you never had to spend another penny on a weight loss gimmick again? This book was written to help you achieve the best health of your life, as well as, to draw closer to God. God does not want you going around the same mountain, time and time again. He wants you free. 2 Cor. 3:17 says, *"Where the spirit of the Lord is, there is liberty,"* and beloved, I want you to experience that liberty.

For more than half of my life, I tried to change just about everything about myself.

I felt I was too fat, too hippy, too loud, too soft-spoken, too ugly, too conservative, too black, too easy, too afraid, too lazy, too worldly, too Godly, and most of all, too undisciplined to make any of these changes stick. Talk about bondage!

Not until I cried out like Paul in Romans 7:24 to be delivered from this body of death did I begin to receive God's healing, peace and rest from all the stories I was telling myself. It's an incredible feeling of rest to be able to do less and receive more. My prayer is that you will receive the same.

The process of God gently changing me continues day by day, bit by bit. I want to share with you what God has taught me to so far. I pray that you receive it and allow it to shape you into the precious miracle that God has created you to be.

I love you and pray for your victory.

Cathy Morenzie

Additional Resources

Over the years I've created additional resources to help people get the most out of these principals or in response to what people continually asked me for and about. All of the following are completely optional but each will, in it's own way, help you to get more from the following 21 days of learning about Weight Loss, God's Way.

Weight Loss, God's Way Challenge

Originally a Facebook Support Group to help women to complete this book, our Challenge has become even more popular than my books. Includes a private Facebook group, daily emails and short, funny but profound daily video messages that really help to convey how each principal shows up in our day to day weight loss journey. Best of all - it's free.

www.weightlossgodswaybonus.com

Healthy by Design: 21 Day Meal Plan

Even though we don't discuss diet in *Weight Loss, God's Way*, I was continually asked by people in our on-line Challenge about what foods to eat or not eat and why. Seeing the confusion around what's comprises a healthy diet and knowing many people wanted to see results quickly, I created a meal plan to go along with the 21 days of this book to address both of those issues. It includes nutrition information, shopping lists and over 60 delicious recipes that will help you to lose weight in a healthy nutritious and often delicious way.

Healthy by Design: Reflections of God's Love

While *Weight Loss, God's Way* was and is, the introduction to these biblical weight loss principals, *Reflections* is as it's name suggestions, a deeper, more matured look back on how God's love and grace has benefitted the many thousands of people touched by them. Includes 21 days of devotions, prayers, quotes from woman who've taken the challenge, declarations, mediations and reflection exercises, even a daily song to celebrate God's love in our lives.

21 DAYS
GOD'S
WAY

DAY 1 – WHAT'S YOUR GOAL?

Scripture Reflection:

"The plans of the diligent lead to profit as surely as haste leads to poverty." ~ Proverbs 21:5 NIV

"Failing to plan, is planning to fail." ~ Benjamin Franklin

So you're ready to start your weight loss journey, congratulations! Before you can start, do you know what you want? Do you know how long it will take you to reach your goal? Your goal will begin to come to fruition only when you are clear on what you want. Writing down your goal sends out a clear message to yourself and the world about who you are and what you are capable of completing.

As you write down your goals, you will begin to align your will with your heavenly Father's. To become crystal clear on your goals, they must be specific, measurable, attainable, realistic and time-constrained (S.M.A.R.T).

It's highly likely that you've set goals many times before and have had limited levels of success. So why will it be different this time? Read the story of Nehemiah and apply his success principles to your weight loss.

We learn in the book of Nehemiah that he (Nehemiah) had an 'impossible' goal; yet through constant prayer combined with preparation and planning, he was able to make the impossible possible. Our response needs to be as Nehemiah's when we are confronted with an overwhelming goal.

Before attempting to do anything, Nehemiah 'mourned, fasted and prayed to the God of heaven.'(Neh. Ch 1:4b) In fact, we read that he prayed spontaneously at least 8 times. He had a clear and specific goal with clear timelines.

Today's Health Challenge

In the space below record exactly what you want. How much weight do you want/need to lose? Write it out in a much detail as you can.

Workspace/Reflections:

Today's Confession:

Thank you for giving me wisdom to set realistic goals that glorify you. I submit my goals and plans to you and I trust you to show me the way. I bring my goals in alignment with your will and purpose for my life. I declare that my goals will come to fruition. I am successful and victorious in the name of Jesus.

DAY 2 - COUNT THE COSTS - WHAT ARE YOU WILLING TO DO?

Scripture Reflection:

> *"If any man will come after me...."* ~ Matt. 16:24

> *"Something happens whenever you sacrifice"* ~ T.D. Jakes

There's no denying that there are mindset differences between thin and healthy people vs. people who struggle to maintain their weight. 'Thin' people see food, their health, their bodies, exercise and life in general from a different perspective than 'overweight' people. They make definite and distinct CHOICES and are willing to make sacrifices that most others don't. So the real question for the person trying to lose weight becomes, 'How much are you willing to do?' If weight release is something you really want then get ready to make the necessary changes to make it happen.

- Are you willing to make the time for exercise regardless of how you feel?
- Are you willing to eat only when you're hungry and stop when you're full?
- Are you willing to eat for health and not for pleasure?
- Are you willing to pay the price?
- Are you willing to accept that you are 100% responsible for your weight release?
- Are you willing to go for counselling or commit to additional support that you might need to overcome your blockages?

The famous 'wall of fame' in Hebrews 11 is a perfect example of people in the bible who overcame the odds and pushed past their comfort level to do what they were called to do. Noah subjected himself to ridicule of his entire community to build a huge boat on dry land. (Gen 6:1-11:32) At God's command, Abraham sacrificed his comfortable life as he knew it to journey to a strange and foreign land (Genesis 12:1).

15

There are countless other stories of heroes who made incredible sacrifices such as Gideon (Judges 6-8), Samson (Judges 13:24-16:31), David (1 Samuel 16, 1 Kings 2), Daniel (Daniel 6), Paul (Acts 7:58-28:31), Samuel (1 Samuel 1-28) and all the prophets.

The fact is, success at anything will take sacrifice and hard work. It will require that you make up your mind that you want to change; no matter what. Yes, change is scary and your body and mind will fight against change but know that God understands your fears, your weaknesses and your disappointments and will never give you more than you can bear. (1 Cor. 10:13)

Today's Health Challenge

Share what adjustments you are going to make to reach your goal.

Workspace/Reflections:

Today's Confession:

I am as bold as a lion. I can endure to the end because you are my strength and shield. I have the capacity for victorious living. I operate in excellence and purpose to complete every task that I set out to do. I can do all things through Christ who gives me strength.

DAY 3 - COUNT THE COST-
THE CONSEQUENCES OF INACTION

Scripture Reflection:

"If you keep quite at a time like this, deliverance and relief for the Jews will arise from some other place, but you and your relatives will die." ~ Esther 4:14

"Those who think they have no time for bodily exercise will sooner or later have to find time for illness." ~ Edward Stanley

Yesterday we looked at some of the sacrifices and costs associated with reaching your weight release goals but have you ever thought about the costs associated with not reaching your goal? What will happen if you don't stop your poor eating habits? Your lack of physical activity? If you don't stop consuming so much sugar, fat and calories? What will it cost your family? What will the cost be to your self-esteem? Your relationships? Your joy?

It's difficult to take a long hard look at all the costs of unfulfilled goals and desires. Sometimes the pain is so hard to face that we would much rather hide our head in the sand, than face the truth about how much pain we are causing ourselves. However, until we confront the pain that we are costing ourselves and others, we will never be motivated enough to want to move past it.

In the book of Esther we see a woman faced with a difficult decision. Although she was a queen and enjoyed the benefits of the king's power and wealth, her position came with a price. She could have lived a comfortable life in a palace with a king but the costs meant jeopardizing the safety of the entire Jewish race. An entire race may not be dependent on your weight loss but then again the legacy of health that you leave for your family might be. Will you leave them a legacy of blessings or curses?

17

Today's Health Challenge

Throughout the day today, complete the statement below. Write out at least seven different answers. Try your best to record them as you think about them instead of trying to remember at the end of the day. Reflect on your feelings as your day progresses.

<u>*Workspace/Reflections:*</u>

The cost if I don't release the weight is...
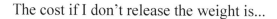

The cost if I don't release the weight is...

The cost if I don't release the weight is...

Today's Confession:

All things work together for good. My pain will turn in to laughter, my cross will be exchanged for a crown and my mourning will be turned into dancing. I am blessed and I am a blessing. My disappointments of the past will be turned into testimonies in the name of Jesus.

DAY 4 - UNDERSTANDING THE PROCESS – LITTLE BY LITTLE

Scripture Reflection:

"Little by little I will drive them out before you, until you have increased enough to take possession of the land." ~ Exodus 23:30

"Take the first step in faith. You don't have to see the whole staircase, just take the first step." ~ Martin Luther King Jr.

How many years did it take you to gain your excess weight? Even though it may have taken you many years to gain weight, we tend to want to lose weight quickly.

Programs like the 'Biggest Loser' have created the illusion that weight loss is quick. They show people losing twenty-five pounds in a week. However, the fast track is never the right path. Change comes through renewing your mind daily with the Word of God. It's a process that happens day by day, little by little, step by step, from glory to glory. God's goal is Christ's fullness in our life. He wants to bring us to new levels and allow us to experience a life of freedom from all the things that keep us bound.

As the Israelites marched out of Egypt, through the Red Sea, and into the wilderness, God promised he would be with them through the entire journey. He also promised that he would help them have victory over all of their enemies and was very specific on how he would help them. God says, "I will drive them out little by little until you have increased enough to take possession of the land." (Exodus 23:30) Why would an all powerful God take his time to act? God understands that to be victorious, certain skills must be developed such as persistence, patience, strategy, and submission. These qualities are not developed overnight. God wants us to get the lessons as well as the blessings. Success comes step by step.

Are you also prepared to take it step by step, little by little?

19

Today's Health Challenge:

How long will it you to reach your goal weight? (Assume 1-2 pounds per week) Be sure to adjust for set-backs and unforeseen circumstances.

Workspace/Reflections:

Today's Confession:

Thank you for your promises. I am making progress. From victory to victory, success to success, I am getting stronger each day. I am more than an over-comer. I am unstoppable and I am advancing in everything I put my mind to. I am unstoppable!

DAY 5 - SUBMIT TO GOD

Scripture Reflection:

"The LORD went before them by day in a pillar of cloud to lead them along the way, and by night in a pillar of fire to give them light" ~ Exodus13:21-22

"You cannot fulfill God's purposes for your life while focusing on your own plans." ~ Rick Warren, The Purpose Driven Life

Just what does it mean to you to submit your weight loss program to God? Do you even know what it looks like? Being open to His leading and prompting? Admitting to Him your inability to do it without Him? Inviting Him to partner with you? Hearing only what He is telling you through your journal entries and prayer time? These are all practical forms of submission.

If we could lose weight (or rid ourselves of any other stumbling block) on our own, then, we would not need God. Strong willpower, self-discipline, and self-control may help you reach your goal, but chances are that the journey will not be enjoyable, and definitely not sustainable. Instead of always getting frustrated trying to do it your way and wasting time, money and your health; the first and most important step is to submit your weight loss program to God.

God gives us a beautiful illustration of how he wants us to live with Him. From the time of the exodus until the Israelites entered the Promised Land, the Lord led them by day with a pillar of cloud, and by night with a pillar of fire. God is just as faithful to us if we allow him to lead. It may not be clouds and fire – for us it may be that still small voice, the confirmation from a friend or the inner feeling of peace. He also promises us that He will never leave us or forsake us.

You CAN rest from all of your efforts; no more crazy diets or gimmicks; no more wasted money, no more frustration, and no more guilt or condemnation. Starting today, refuse to take another step in your health program without God.

Cathy Morenzie

Today's Health Challenge

What conscious behaviors and actions are you currently engaging in that show your lack of submission in the area of your weight loss process. List 5-10 of them below and then begin asking the Holy Spirit to help you. Say each one of them aloud one by one.

Workspace/Reflections:

Today's Confession:

I walk in your presence today and I choose to honor you God today by what I eat, and in all I do. I submit my weight, my health and my body to you. I walk with courage, discipline and perseverance in times of testing and temptation. I am blessed and prosperous in You.

22

DAY 6 - THE POWER OF PRAYER

Scripture Reflection:

"Pray so that you will not fall into temptation." ~ Luke 22:39

"Pray more, worry less"

Is it really necessary to bring prayer into your weight loss program? Obviously, yes! Most people today want to lose weight. Many people pay good money to lose weight. Yet most people are still struggling with a weight issue.

Hands down, prayer is the most effective and precious gift that God has given us. It is an intimate time of communication with God. God himself invites us to request what we need and then trust Him to meet our needs.

The power of prayer is life-changing. The more we reach out to God in prayer, the more we experience His transforming peace. Through prayer we war against our strongholds, we replace our fear with faith and we receive his peace when nothing around us is peaceful. Through prayer God's power gets downloaded into us.

Jesus asked the disciples to pray so that they would not fall into temptation. (Luke 22:39) He knew that they were going to face many difficulties and wanted them to be proactive. After Jesus instructed them, he then walked away from them and prayed on his own. As he prayed verse 43 says that 'an angel from heaven appeared and strengthened him.'

Imagine praying and immediately being strengthened to continue on your journey. The same God that strengthened Jesus in the garden is the same God that will strengthen you in all your journeys. Trust him today to meet your needs by spending time in prayer with him. God always delivers on his promises!

Today's Health Challenge

Prayer is one of our greatest weapons to war against the enemy, to align our will's with God's and to help us to resist temptations. Based on where you currently are in your walk, this may or may not be an overwhelming exercise for you. Your health challenge today is to boldly say your prayer out loud. You can do it in the mirror or wherever you feel comfortable.

Workspace/Reflections:

Today's Confession:

I thank you that we don't have to be worried or anxious about anything. We bring our request to you with thanksgiving and stand in confidence that You will bring it to fruition. We submit our request to You and are able to do exceeding abundantly above all that we can ask or think.

DAY 7 - THE POWER OF CHOICE

Scripture Reflection:

"Give yourselves completely to God, for you were dead, but now you have a new life" ~ Rom. 6:13

"You are free to make whatever choice you want but you are not free from the consequences of the choice" ~ unknown

In order for change to be permanent God wants us to replace our old patterns and behaviors with new ways of being. These new behaviors must be continually applied until they are consistent and habitual in your life otherwise when we feel afraid and vulnerable we will revert back to what we've always done.

Change will require the perfect blend of faith and action. (2 Samuel 10:12) Once you've submitted your weight release to God, he will prompt you to move to higher levels of success in this area and all other areas of your life. What is the Holy Spirit prompting you to change first? There are probably a whole lot of areas where you feel you need to change. Identify them and choose one that you are going to commit to changing immediately.

Get up....Go…Grow! God called the Israelites to move from their present state of slavery to a life of freedom. Their journey was fraught with many challenges, and through them all, the Israelites went back to what they knew best – grumbling, complaining, living in disobedience and worshipping false idols.

The result-- 40 years of wandering aimlessly for a journey scholars estimate would take anywhere from eleven days to one year! Glory to God that He has given us a new heart and a new spirit that allows us to live by his rules and not our own (Ezekiel 36:26-27).

Today's Health Challenge

Take some time and find a scripture you will recite to 'renew your mind' every time you don't stick to your goal. As you make a daily choice to stay focused on your goal, God will honour your commitment and strengthen you on the journey.

Workspace/Reflections:

Today's Confession:

I am dead to sin. Your strength and grace has changed me and renewed me. I have a new life in you and do things that lead to holiness and joy. The power of your life-giving spirit has freed me from the power of sin. Your spirit that controls my mind has given me life and peace.

DAY 8 - SPEAKING TO YOUR SITUATION - POWERFUL POSITIVE AFFIRMATIONS

Scripture Reflection:

"The tongue has the power of life and death" ~ Proverbs 18:21

"The greatest discovery of my generation is that human beings can alter their lives by altering their attitudes of mind."
~ William James

Affirmations is one of the most powerful tools God has given us to combat every single problem in our lives! The book of John starts off, "In the beginning was the Word." Huh? What does that mean? In Hebrew scripture, the Word was an agent of creation. So powerful that Psalm 33:6 states that, "the Lord merely spoke, and the heavens were created."

Is it possible that God has also given us this same power? Then God said, "Let us make man in our image, to be like ourselves." (Gen. 1:26) This includes the power to speak to our situations and circumstances …you could say to this mountain, 'Move from here to there,' (Matt. 17:20) and it would move.

Speak the Word of God over your life. When Jesus was being tempted in the desert his greatest weapon was the Word of God. Three times Satan came at him from different angles and all three times Jesus spoke the Word of God. He acknowledged that man shall not live by bread alone but by every word that proceeds out of the mouth… What we say can give us life.

God gives us guidelines for how to powerfully use declarations:

- Always declare in the positive- I am strong and courageous
- Be clear and specific- (James 1:6)
- Believe (Matt 17:20)
- Say them out loud (Psalms 119:13)
- Say them consistently- memorize them (Psalm 119:9, 11)
- Don't beg or ask but boldly declare (Proverbs 28:1)

Today's Health Challenge

In your journal or using an electronic device, record how often you catch yourself saying something negative about yourself. Write out a powerful affirmation today using the 6 points listed above. Memorize it and recite it throughout the day.

Workspace/Reflections:

Today's Confession:

I have the faith to move mountains. The Holy Spirit in me has made the impossible possible. I am more than a conqueror and I can overcome any obstacle that stands in my path. No weapon formed against me shall prosper. I am constantly making progress. I am a success.

DAY 9 – RAISE YOUR AWARENESS

Scripture Reflection:

"Do not conform any longer to the pattern of this world, but be transformed by the renewing of your mind." ~ Romans 12:2

"Let us not look back in anger, nor forward in fear, but around in awareness."~ James Thurber

Do you often just go with the flow of life? Are you making things happen in life or is life happening to you? If we are truly honest with ourselves, much of our lives happen to us. We live on automatic pilot and accept the hand that life has dealt us. We are often not in control of the food choices we make. We grab something fast because we are in a rush, we eat because we have a craving for something, or someone gives us something to eat and we are too polite to say no.

This level of living keeps us stuck and robs us of our joy. Your successful weight loss will require you to tune in to all the choices you make, your thought patterns, your motivation for doing what you do and even to evaluate your decision making process.

In the book of Daniel; Daniel, Hananiah, Mishael and Azariah were faced with a dilemma where demands were placed on them. They were taken from their homeland and were told to eat food that was not part of their lifestyle or their custom. But Daniel and his friends resolved that they would not eat the King's food. They had the Lord on their side and if we allow Him into our lives, so do we. Like Daniel, we must resolve to obey God rather than the pressures of this world. From Daniel, we also learn that we must have a plan in place to resist temptation before it arises. He was determined to stay committed to his principles and choices.

In the New Testament book of Romans, we also learn the difference between living consciously by focusing our life on Jesus versus living under the Law of Moses which was ritualistic and only provided temporary relief. Romans 8:5 teaches us that, "those who are dominated by the sinful nature think about sinful things, but those who are controlled by the

Holy Spirit think about things that please the Spirit."

Today's Health Challenge

Today you will be 100% conscious of everything you put into your mouth. You will only eat foods that will build your body and not cause it any harm. This will take some additional planning on your part so take some time before you leave the house to organize yourself. Avoid all processed foods, all fast foods, all additives and preservatives, all sugar and caffeine.

Workspace/Reflections:

Today's Confession:

I love you Lord and thank you for your spirit that lives in me. My mind is set on things above. I become more and more like you each day. I am created in your image. I make responsible choices and decisions. I have the ability to solve my problems with you as my guide. I take authority over this day in the Name of Jesus.

DAY 10 - WHAT'S STOPPING YOU?

Scripture Reflection:

"I do the things I don't want to do but the things I want to do those I don't do." ~ Romans 7:15

"Character is expressed through our behavior patterns, or natural responses to things." ~ Joyce Meyer

Why is it that in spite of our deep desire for weight loss, we continually make the same mistakes of poor food choices, and other disempowering behaviors? Why do we continue to cling so tenaciously to patterns that don't serve us?

Truth is most of our patterns are unconscious. We've held on to them so long that we don't even realize that they keep us stuck. To finally be free of the things that hold us back we must first identify our defeating patterns, behaviors, thoughts and choices and turn them over to God. These 'dream-robbers' keep us from living the life that we were born to live. Our assignment is to subdue and over-come these dream-robbers if we want to keep unwanted weight off forever.

Paul's struggle with sin was as real for him as it is for us. In Romans 7:15 we hear the cry of a desperate man so frustrated with his sin nature.

In Luke 4:8, Simon Peter also comes to grips with his sinful nature as he realizes that God is even interested in helping him catch fish! He remarks, "Depart from me, for I am a sinful man, O Lord!"

Coming to grips with our sinful nature is the first step in allowing the Spirit of God to dwell richly in you, gradually replacing your fears and faults with Christ's freedom from what's been holding you back. Like Simon Peter (and Paul), once we realize our sinful nature and understand how deeply its engrained in us, then and only then, can we begin to understand that Christ is the only one that can help us once we are willing to allow Him.

Today's Health Challenge

Write out one recurrent pattern or behavior that keeps you from reaching your goal. Now write out how these behaviors have showed up in your life at the following stages:

Workspace/Reflections:

Childhood:

Teenager:

Adult:

Today's Confession:

Have mercy on me Christ. You have searched me God and helped me uncover my anxious thoughts. I now begin the process of rooting them out forever. I thank you for replacing my old behaviors with new ones that are pleasing in your eyes. Because of your love I am dead to sin. I boldly take hold of your power that gives me victory over sin.

DAY 11 - WHAT DO YOU BELIEVE?

Scripture Reflection:

"They continued to follow their own gods according to the religious customs of the nations from which they came."
~ 2 Kings 18:33

"Growth demands a temporary surrender of security. It may mean giving up familiar but limiting patterns, safe but unrewarding work, values no longer believed in, and relationships that have lost their meaning." ~ John C. Maxwell

We all have things that we believe about ourselves. We may have been told them or we may have internalized a belief as a result of something that's happened to us in our childhood. In relation to our health, some of these beliefs might sound something like this:

- 'God is not concerned about the physical, its what's inside that counts'
- 'Physical exercise profits little;'
- 'Realistically, chances are I'll never be thin;'
- 'I'll put all the weight back on again if I lose it anyway;'

These beliefs or positions about life can sometimes get in the way of us reaching our goals. As we unconsciously carry these beliefs with us into adulthood, they often sabotage our plans and goals. These faulty beliefs impact our emotions, our actions and our health. Breakthrough will require a change in these thought patterns.

In the book of 2 Kings, the Israelites begin their slippery slope into idolatry. Their desire was to serve God but their actions led to idolatry and corruption. The king of Assyria saw first-hand how harshly God dealt with idolatry so he sent for priests to teach the Israelites how to worship the Lord. The problem was that the new settlers also continued to worship their own gods according to the religious customs of the nations from which they came. The result—their ruin.

Israel was conquered because it refused to focus on the one true God.

They could not turn away from their old beliefs even though it led them away from God. What beliefs are you refusing to let go of? Understand the cost of holding on… It's not worth it.

Over the next few days we will look at how our beliefs make us engage in unhealthy behaviours such as excuse-making, blaming, procrastinating and emotional eating. We do them because they protect us from the pain of these deep rooted beliefs. Noticing which ones you engage in is a big first step towards freedom.

Today's Health Challenge

For today's challenge. Identify a limiting belief that sabotages your weight loss efforts.

Workspace/Reflections:

Today's Confession:

Your promises are for eternity. Every generational curse and everything spoken against my health is broken in the Name of Jesus. I declare that I am in sound health in my body, mind and spirit. I am strong and coura- geous and successful in everything I do. I meditate on your word day and night. Him, who the Son sets free, is free indeed and I declare my freedom in you.

DAY 12 - REASONS OR RESULTS - EXCUSE MAKING

Scripture Reflection:

"I have no one to help me into the pool when the water is stirred. While I am trying to get in, someone else goes down ahead of me."
~ John 5:7

"He that is good for making excuses is seldom good for anything else." ~ Benjamin Franklin

I can't lose weight because I don't have the time… I can't afford it… I can't afford a gym membership right now… My kids need me… Do any of these sound familiar?

I took a course a few years ago and the facilitator made a powerful statement. He said "in life there are reasons and results—if you have a reason, then you did not get the result." So which would you prefer, a good reason or a good result?

Excuse making is one of the faulty patterns that keep us stuck. Excuses keep us from taking responsibility for our lives and our health. They rob us of our personal power and leave us feeling helpless to our circumstances.

Excuses in and of themselves are just the symptoms of an underlying problem. One of the most important steps in releasing excess weight is to uproot excuse-making and begin dealing with the real issues behind the excuses you make. It's impossible to change what you don't acknowledge.

There's a sad story in the book of John about a man that allowed his infirmity to become his way of life for 38 years! The story outlines a lame man waiting at a healing pool that was believed to heal whoever was the first person to step into the water after it was stirred by an angel of the Lord. (John 5: 1-9) Although he may have had a legitimate excuse (like most of us) for not going after what he wanted, he blamed his situation on other people not helping him. He complained that other people were always jumping ahead of him and that's why he could not receive his healing.

What reasons do you have for why you have not received a breakthrough in this area? As legitimate as our excuses may be, God wants us to take 100% responsibility for our actions and he has equipped us with the ability to do so.

Today's Health Challenges

Make a list of all the excuses (even the legitimate ones) you use to justify why you are not at your ideal, healthy weight.

Workspace/Reflections:

Today's Confession:

Father, you've clothed me with strength and honor; you've empowered me to be strong and courageous. I reclaim my power in You by taking 100% responsibility for our thoughts and actions. I am blessed with the Holy Ghost to accomplish my weight loss goals. I will have a testimony in the Name of Jesus.

DAY 13 - THE BLAME GAME

Scripture Reflection:

"It was the woman who you gave me who gave me the fruit, and I ate it." ~ Gen. 3:12

"I'm only going to stand before God and give an account for my life, not for somebody else's life. If I have a bad attitude, then I need to say there's no point in me blaming you for what's wrong in my life." ~ Joyce Meyer

A close friend to excuse making is the blame game. In this game, you lose no matter how well you play. The blame game sounds something like this: "my husband/wife does the shopping so I have no control of what food is in the house"; "It's my genetics". In this game you are the poor victim and someone else is to blame for why you're overweight. Like excuse-making, ending the blame game will require you to take 100% responsibility for your actions.

The habit of blaming can be seen since the beginning of time. When God asked Adam if he ate the fruit Adam blamed it on the woman. Then when God asked Eve if she ate the forbidden fruit she blamed it on the serpent. As the story plays out we also learn a universal principle that every action will always have a consequence.

As we see in the Garden of Eden, the moment we blame someone else for our actions, we delay our success because we waste time focusing on the wrong problem; we doubt our own abilities to reach our goals; we divert our attention away from the real problem and deprive ourselves of the joy that God has for us. Follow God's plan for your life by refusing to blame anyone or anything for your lack of results.

Today's Health Challenge

Record the names of anyone who you blame for participating directly or indirectly in your not having the ideal health and weight. Take responsibility by apologizing to them today and tell them that effective immediately, you will take 100% percent responsibility for your health.

Workspace/Reflections:

Today's Confession:

Father, forgive me for usurping my responsibility to you for my health and wellness. Excellent health is mine, energy and vitality are mine. I am designed to reach higher levels of health from victory to victory, glory to glory in the name of Jesus!

DAY 14 – AVOIDING PROCRASTINATION

Scripture Reflection:

"How long are you going to wait before taking possession of the remaining land the Lord, the God of your ancestors, has given to you?" ~ Joshua 18:3

"Procrastination may relieve short-term pressure. But it often impedes long-term progress." ~ John Maxwell

Procrastination is another serious barrier that stops us from reaching our goals. It is a lot more complex than just putting things off. A well known psychologist Piers Steel published almost 800 studies on procrastination!

The root cause of procrastination stems from a problem with our relationship with ourselves which directly implies a problem with our relationship with our Heavenly Father. Like many other strongholds, procrastination usually stems from some type of fear: fear of failure; fear of success; fear of being controlled; fear of intimacy; fear of separation and the list can go on and on.

In the Old Testament, Joshua was chosen to be Moses' successor to lead the Israelites to the Promised Land. His greatest strength was his willingness to submit to God. As he assumed his new position, he couldn't help wondering why some of the tribes were procrastinating in possessing the land as God had instructed them. To combat this problem, Joshua took the initiative and delegated three men to take action and move the task forward.

This issue is far too complex to address in this book alone but the Word offers some solutions to get you to start changing this destructive behavior.

First, seek God regarding how to prioritize your schedule (Matt. 6: 33). Then, submit all of our fears to God as you focus on the end result (instead of the fear). See the appendix for scripture to help you combat your fears.

Cathy Morenzie

Today's Health Challenges

What is one main thing that you have been putting off in relation to your weight loss? What big step will you take today to break this spirit of pro-crastination? Record it below.

Workspace/Reflections:

Today's Confession:

I seek your kingdom above all else. I put you before my agendas, my timelines and my priorities. I walk in faith and not fear. I walk in power, victory and a sound mind. I do everything on time and in order. All my steps are ordered by you.

DAY 15 – OVERCOMING EMOTIONAL EATING

Scripture Reflection:

"In your anger do not sin... Do not let the sun go down while you are still angry, and do not give the devil a foothold."
~ Eph. 4: 26-27

"Feel your feelings, don't feed them"

Another destructive behavior that will always sabotage your weight loss program is emotional eating. Experts estimate that 75% of overeating is caused by emotions. Emotional eating is when we eat in response to our feelings regardless of whether we're hungry or not and/or when we use food as a tool or coping mechanism to either numb pain or to feel better. Common feelings that lead to emotional eating include boredom, stress (financial, relational, mental, etc.), loneliness, tiredness and frustration.

In Ephesians 4, Paul teaches how to effectively deal with the stresses of life. He is talking more specifically about strife between people but it also applies to dealing with our inner turmoil. He points out that it's okay to be angry (or experience other emotions) but we must find Godly ways of dealing with it. Unresolved issues give way to the devil operating in our lives. The psalmist also tells us when we are angry to search our hearts and be silent (Psalms 4:4).

But the one thing that Jesus wants above all else is that you spend time listening to him, "sitting at his feet," as it were. That needs to come first, before all these other things. That is where peace is found.

Over time you will learn how to develop appropriate and effective ways of dealing with your emotions such as:

- Take the time to ask yourself what the underlying feeling is that is triggering the emotion
- Submit that feeling/situation over to God – ask Him to handle it instead of food;

- Pause - emotional eating can be so intense but if you can hold off for 10-15 minutes the craving will often subside

Today's Health Challenge:

What emotion led you to eat unnecessarily the last time? What was the underlying feeling?

Workspace/Reflections:

Today's Confession:

Him who the Son sets free is free indeed! I rejoice because I am free from bondage. I am free from emotional eating. I am free to be me, created in your image and destined for greatness. I have the capacity to effectively deal with every situation and circumstance that my mind, people or the enemy will throw my way.

DAY 16 - ARE YOU A GIANT OR A GRASSHOPPER? – POOR SELF-IMAGE

Scripture Reflection:

> *"We even saw giants there, the descendants of Anak. Next to them we felt like grasshoppers...!" ~ Numbers 13:33.*

> *"See yourself as God sees you."*

How do you see yourself when you look in the mirror? Do you focus on your strengths or do your eyes hone in on all the flaws. If we're honest with ourselves, most of us focus on all that's wrong with ourselves rather than on what's right.

Poor self-image one of the big dream robbers. They can be the cause of procrastination, excuse-making, blaming, lack of faith and lack of self-control to name just a few. It will affect how you see the world and how you think the world views you.

In the story in the book of Numbers, ten men were sent to scout out land that God had promised the Israelites. The men returned with fearful stories of giants that would surely devour them even though their reports conflicted with Joshua and Calebs'—two men with great vision and self-esteem. The ten men had such low regard for themselves that they saw themselves as grasshoppers in comparison to their enemies. If you see yourself as small or incapable or not worthy then that's exactly what the world will reflect back to you.

Here's a biblical plan from this story to help you build your self-esteem:

- Believe what God says about you and what He has promised you regardless of what the majority of people (society, friends, and peers) might say about you.
- Have the right attitude - Caleb trusted God to give Israel the land He promised them
- Stand firm and declare positive affirmations to combat negative ones. Caleb declared 'We can certainly conquer it!' (Num. 13:30)

- Learn to distinguish God's voice - God will never condemn you or make you feel bad.
- When the Holy Spirit convicts you of sin, He will always direct you toward a specific action that you can take. (John 3:19-21)

Today's Health Challenge

Write down 10 things that you like about yourself. Choose 1 or 2 scriptures that reveal spiritual truths about who you are in God's eyes.

Workspace/Reflections:

Today's Confession:

I am fearfully and wonderfully made. I am the apple of your eye. There is no condemnation for those who are in Christ Jesus, because through Christ Jesus the spirit set me free from the power of sin and I can certainly conquer this stronghold and any other one that will come my way in your matchless Name!

DAY 17 – STAY SELF-CONTROLLED

Scripture Reflection:

"Be self-controlled and alert. Your enemy the devil prowls around like a roaring lion looking for someone to devour." ~ 1 Peter 5:8

"I have learned that I really do have discipline, self-control, and patience. But they were given to me as a seed, and it's up to me to choose to develop them." ~ Joyce Meyer

On top of the unconscious patterns that can sabotage us, we also engage in many conscious patterns. Lack of control is the first of these behaviors that we will delve into.

We live in a world of extremes. Going without food or overeating both cause us to lose focus and control. Avoid the extremes in life. Popular 12-step programs caution against H.A.L.T. – don't allow yourself to get too hungry, angry, lonely or tired. Extremes wear us out and inhibit our decision-making ability. Poor food choices are often made when we are so tired that our body craves an instant pick-me-up, which is usually unhealthy.

We learn from King David how lack of self-control can lead us into deeper and deeper sin. The book of Samuel 2:11 opens with the subtle but powerful indictment of King David. It reads, 'In the Spring of the year, when kings normally go out to war, David sent Joab and the Israelite army to fight the Ammonites.' Here we learn that prior to falling into sin with Bathsheba, David chose to hang out idly at home with his thoughts instead of going to war with the other soldiers. We should ask ourselves the same question, 'Are we operating in our purpose' and if not, is that causing us to lose our focus and control?

Another example can be found in the New Testament. We learn what happens when we make ourselves too busy. We learn that Martha is gently corrected by Jesus for busying herself in the kitchen and stressing herself out, while Mary's choice to sit at Jesus' feet and listen to him teach is affirmed. (Luke 10:38-42) "'Martha, Martha,' the Lord answered, 'you are worried and upset about many things....'" (10:41)

God's solution for staying self-controlled is found in 1 Peter 5:9. It warns us to be attuned to when we may be vulnerable. Peter also encourages us to be strong in our faith which means that during times of crisis, trials and temptations, we should seek other Christians for support. James gives us another strategy which is to 'humble ourselves before God. Resist the devil and he will flee.' (James 4:7)

Today's Health Challenge:

Record times when you feel vulnerable and out of control. Under what circumstances do you experience this most often? What will be your strategy the next time it happens? Call, text, or email someone in the midst of one of these circumstances today and have them pray with you. (Let them know ahead of time so they will be ready)

Workspace/Reflections:

Today's Confession:

I stand firm against the enemy and he flees. I keep my eyes fixed on you God because You are the author and perfecter of my faith. I stand firm in Your word. It is my sword and my shield. Your word is a light unto my feet and a light unto my path. It brings me comfort, protection and strength in times of need.

DAY 18 - HOW TO STAY FOCUSED

Scripture Reflection:

"...knew you not that I must be about my Father's business?"
~ Luke 2:49

"When trouble comes, focus on God's ability to care for you."
~ Charles Stanley

It's so easy for us to get distracted, emotional, discouraged, or just plain tired. How do we maintain our focus when we don't feel like it? It's so easy to lose our focus. We live in a society where we have so many demands placed on us; there's little time for rest or reflection and we really don't know how to function when we don't have 10 things on the go.

In the bible we see a sharp contrast between how Jesus stayed focused and how his disciples were constantly distracted. In the popular story of Peter's attempt to walk on water we can learn a lot about focus. Peter started off well—he was actually doing it! Then Peter experienced the same issue many of us experience.

He took his eye off his goal and focused on the overwhelming situation. The result—he sank. If we focus on the challenges and magnitude of weight release then we will also sink in despair. To stay focused on your weight loss goal when situations are difficult; focus on the power of the Holy Spirit rather than on your own weaknesses. (2 Cor. 12:9)

Jesus teaches us a lot about focus. What action steps can you incorporate from Jesus' life to keep you from getting distracted?

- Jesus often went away on his own to refocus and spend time with his Father. (Mark 1:35, Luke 5:16, Matt 26:39)
- Jesus used scripture to counter the attacks of Satan. (Matt. 4:1-11)
- Jesus resolved to stay the course regardless of the circumstances. (Luke 9:51)
- Jesus enlisted help and support of others. (Luke 10:1)

Today's Health Challenge

Write out the main things that cause you to lose focus of your weight loss goal.

Workspace/Reflections:

Today's Confession:

I have the mind of Christ. My mind is set on the spirit which is life and peace. My mind is being renewed day by day. The Holy Spirit lives in me and quickens me to do His will.

DAY 19 - PARTNERSHIPS

Scripture Reflection:

"He who walks with wise men will be wise, but the companion of fools will be destroyed." ~ Proverbs 13:30

"Accountability breeds response-ability." ~ Stephen Covey

Weight loss challenges tend to be a very isolating and lonely stronghold. No one wants their friends, family and loved ones to know how much they're struggling so people tend to isolate themselves and try to solve their problems on their own. Like many other strongholds, weight releasing is not a journey that you should even attempt to do on your own.

As you go through challenges, you will need others around you who will motivate you, help build your integrity, show you how loved and cherished you are, give you a different perspective that you may be able to see on your own, and create a hedge of protection around you. Your partner will also give you the encouragement you need when you're unable to motivate yourself.

When you're down or frustrated, it's natural to call someone who will make you feel better. This person will usually offer you some encouragement and pump you up. This type of accountability is great but it's not always the best thing for us. Sometimes we need counsel that will lovingly advise us that we were wrong, that we are being immature or that we need to repent for our behaviors. In the bible, Nathan was one such wise man. He knew that he had to confront David about his sin. He knew that the truth would hurt so he had to come up with creative ways of showing him that he was wrong without getting David's back up. (2 Sam.12) It took great courage and tact to speak to David in a way that would get him to see his mistakes. Your accountability partners should be able to speak to you in such a way.

Surround yourself with someone who loves you enough to correct you and wants you to succeed. Begin to pray that God would show you who your accountability partner should be. Having an accountability partner will require a high level of transparency and honesty.

Be vulnerable, honest and willing to hear what your accountability partner has to say. The truth sometimes hurts. No one likes facing their 'dark side' or feeling like their 'stuff 'is being exposed but trust that these steps are beneficial for your growth and eventual victory.

Today's Health Challenge

In the space below, write down all the people who will be supporting you on this journey.

Workspace/Reflections:

Today's Confession:

I confess my sins to another as you have instructed. I thank you for my partner and I thank you that we are able to sharpen each other. As iron sharpens iron, we sharpen each other. We stand in agreement to manifest what you have already done in heaven right here on earth!

DAY 20 - MAKING YOU A PRIORITY

Scripture Reflection:

"You expected much, but see, it turned out to be little...Because of my house, which remains a ruin, while each of you is busy with his own house." ~ Haggai 1:9

"Well-ordered self-love is right and natural." ~ Thomas Aquinas

What do you think is the #1 reason people give for not exercising? If you said 'time' you are 100% correct and it may also be your #1 reason for not exercising and taking care of yourself as you should. The problem is not really an issue of time (or lack of it) but rather an issue of values - what is truly important to you?

We give our time and attention to what we deem important to us. We say we want to lose weight but more often than not, this goal gets bumped to the bottom of our 'to-do' list. So the real question becomes, 'How important is losing weight to you'? Even though most of us would say it's very important, we're so 'stuck' in our current routine that it's impossible to see how we could possibly fit anything else into the day.

In his book, *'The Purpose Driven Life'*, best-selling author Rick Warren teaches us that we have just enough time to do what God's called us to do and if you can't get it all done, it means you're trying to do more than God intended. Are there things in your life that take up too much of your time and don't leave you time to do the things you really want? Then it's time to take stock of what you really want and begin to reshape your schedule to make it a priority.

In the book of Haggai we learn an important lesson about prioritizing our time. God had given the Jews an assignment to finish the Temple when they returned from captivity. Like most of us, they got busy, forgot their priorities and grew apathetic to things that were once important to them.

Through Haggai, God challenged them to action, *"'You expected much, but see, it turned out to be little. What you brought home, I blew away.*

Why' declares the LORD Almighty. 'Because of my house, which remains a ruin, while each of you is busy with his own house.'" Haggai 1:8-10. Has God been calling you to rebuild your temple?

Today's Health Challenge

Making you a priority will often mean resetting your priorities by saying no to many other things that are vying for your time. Your goal today is to say 'no' to all requests (non-work related) that are presented to you. Say no to all lunch offers, phone conversations, etc. Practice the art of saying 'no' all day long and share your experience with your accountability partner.

Workspace/Reflections:

Today's Confession:

Father we thank you that when we put You first, you teach us how to prioritize. My steps are ordered by you. I do first things first. I seek your Kingdom above all else and in doing so, You teach me how to make the most of my day. In all I do, I worship You. My time is in Your hands and You have blessed it and given me good success.

DAY 21 - STAYING ON COURSE

Scripture Reflection:

"Whether you turn to the right or to the left, your ears will hear a voice behind you, saying, "This is the way; walk in it.""
~ Isaiah 30:21

"You are the only real obstacle in your path to a fulfilling life."
~ Les Brown

Do you know when you're on the right track? How do you know that this time it's going to work? Morning devotion time; maintaining a food journal; bringing your lunch to work; grocery shopping each week; taking time to plan your day; taking time to exercise.... There are many actions that make us feel like we're on track. They motivate us to stay the course and energize us to persevere for another day. These markers or guideposts are effective tools that keep us on track. Once we follow the guidepost then we are guaranteed to get where we're going.

Don't be afraid to try something new - it might not work but it's okay. Making a poor decision doesn't mean we're forever out of God's will. That's the beauty of Scripture. It contains story after story of people who made bad decisions, but God still uses them mightily. Two examples include: Abraham (Genesis 12:11-13) and David (2 Samuel 11). They both did things that were clearly wrong, but God worked through them to accomplish great achievements. God can use all of our decisions, whether they're right, wrong, or neutral. What's important is that you get on course and listen for God's voice to direct you.

God wants to show you the path that you should follow. He has given us the promise, "My sheep hear My voice." There are many examples of great men and women in the bible who listened for God's voice and then acted as a result. (Hab. 2:2, I Kings 19:12). Like Habakkuk, a good tool for communicating with God is to journal what he is saying to you. Try writing out a question to Him and wait for his response. You can 'test it' once He responds, by searching the scriptures for confirmation.

Today's Health Challenge

In this book, we identified many areas that might be preventing you from reaching your healthy weight. I suggest you spend some time in prayer and ask God how he wants you to proceed. Listen intently for His responses and journal them.

Workspace/Reflections:

Today's Confession:

Thank you that You've promised that you would never leave us or forsake us. You are our teacher and our guide. Your ways are always right and true. I hear Your voice in all I do. Your word guides me in all I do. I fix my eyes upon You and your Spirit gives me direction.

PUTTING IT ALL TOGETHER

I commend you and congratulate your courage and determination to be in the best health and glorify your Father.

You have now laid the groundwork for a deeper and more intimate relationship with your body and with the creator of your body.

Remember that this is just the beginning. There is still much work to do and I encourage you to continue to reach higher heights in the Lord and in your health. Each new level brings new goals, new blessings and a deeper understanding of who you are in Christ.

He created you to be whole and complete. He wants you to lack nothing. He loves you unconditionally and whole-heartedly and He wants you to love yourself the same way. It brings your Father glory when you take care of His temple - its one of His gifts to you.

As a kingdom citizen, rest in the fact that All things have been placed under your feet. You have victory over your weight challenges and every other stronghold that attempts to defeat you. You have been given that authority and now it's time use it.

To effectively exercise your authority, you'll have to study and pray God's word until you are firmly rooted in Him. Develop the new discipline of speaking the Word of God over your weight, your health and your entire life. It will dramatically change you. Use the additional scriptures below to continue to meditate on the Word of God.

I recommend you review this book periodically to help engrain the new habits and track your spiritual growth. Consider adding one of our additional resources (Challenge, Meal Plan or *Reflections* devotional) to gain even more benefit from reviewing these principals.

It is my prayer that these biblical principles to weight loss will lead you to a long life of excellent health, peace, freedom and joy.

Thank You

I'm so delighted that you've not only bought this book, but you've read it through to the end. I pray that these principles have been as much of a blessing to you, as they have been for myself and countless other women around the world.

If you've been blessed by this book (and/or online challenge), then please, dont' keep it a secret!

There are millions of women who need to hear this message. Please take a moment to leave an honest book review so more people can discover this book as well.

I recommend you re-read this book (and/or it's counterpart - Reflections of God's Love) periodically to refresh these concepts and to see how far you've progressed. I pray and hope to meet you in our online Challenge or in our ongoing monthly weight loss support group - Haven.

In Haven I work directly with our members through our private Facebook group, provide weekly lessons, live calls, meal plans, workouts and guest speakers.

To learn more about Haven visit:
www.cathymorenzie.com/membershipprogram

If you'd like to receive my free newsletter with more great spiritual and practical advice for Christian women (and enlightened men) - please subscribe at:
www.cathymorenzie.com

APPENDIX - ADDITIONAL SCRIPTURES

ADDITIONAL SCRIPTURES

DAY 1 - GOAL SETTING

Philippians 3:13-14-Brothers, I do not consider that I have made it my own. But one thing I do: forgetting what lies behind and straining forward to what lies ahead, I press on toward the goal for the prize of the upward call of God in Christ Jesus.

2 Chronicles 15:7-But you, take courage! Do not let your hands be weak, for your work shall be rewarded.

2 Peter 3:18-But grow in the grace and knowledge of our Lord and Savior Jesus Christ. To him be the glory both now and to the day of eternity. Amen.

Philippians 4:12-I know how to be brought low, and I know how to abound. In any and every circumstance, I have learned the secret of facing plenty and hunger, abundance and need.

DAY 2 - COUNT THE COSTS

Hebrews 5:8-Although he was a son, he learned obedience through what he suffered.

Romans 12:1-I appeal to you therefore, brothers, by the mercies of God, to present your bodies as a living sacrifice, holy and acceptable to God, which is your spiritual worship.

2 Corinthians 6:14-Do not be unequally yoked with unbelievers. For what partnership has righteousness with lawlessness? Or what fellowship has light with darkness?

Acts 17:26-And he made from one man every nation of mankind to live on all the face of the earth, having determined allotted periods and the boundaries of their dwelling place…

Cathy Morenzie

DAY 3 - CONSEQUENCES OF INACTION

Proverbs 14:12-There is a way that seems right to a man, but its end is the way to death.

James 4:17-So whoever knows the right thing to do and fails to do it, for him it is sin.

James 4:3-You ask and do not receive, because you ask wrongly, to spend it on your passions.

DAY 4 - UNDERSTANDING THE PROCESS

Proverbs 13:11-Wealth gained hastily will dwindle, but whoever gathers little by little will increase it.

Luke 16:10-One who is faithful in a very little is also faithful in much, and one who is dishonest in a very little is also dishonest in much.

Proverbs 24:27-Prepare your work outside; get everything ready for yourself in the field, and after that build your house.

DAY 5 - SUBMISSION

2 Corinthians 5:17-Therefore, if anyone is in Christ, he is a new creation. The old has passed away; behold, the new has come.

John 14:26-But the Helper, the Holy Spirit, whom the Father will send in my name, he will teach you all things and bring to your remembrance all that I have said to you.

Proverbs 3:6-… in all your ways acknowledge Him and he will make your paths straight.

DAY 6 - POWER OF PRAYER

John 14:14-If you ask me anything in my name, I will do it.

1 John 5:14-15-And this is the confidence that we have toward him, that if we ask anything according to his will he hears us. And if we know that he hears us in whatever we ask, we know that we have the requests that we have asked of him.

James 5:18-Then he prayed again, and heaven gave rain, and the earth bore its fruit.

DAY 7 - MAKING POWERFUL CHOICES

Proverbs 14:12-There is a way that seems right to a man, but its end is the way to death

Matthew 7:13-14-Enter by the narrow gate. For the gate is wide and the way is easy that leads to destruction, and those who enter by it are many. For the gate is narrow and the way is hard that leads to life, and those who find it are few.

Exodus 21:24-25-Eye for eye, tooth for tooth, hand for hand, foot for foot, burn for burn, wound for wound, stripe for stripe.

DAY 8 - POWERFUL AFFIRMATIONS

Psalm 119:13-With my lips I recount all the laws that come from your mouth.

Psalm 40:9-I proclaim righteousness in the great assembly; I do not seal my lips, as you know, O LORD.

Psalm 22:22-I will declare your name to my brothers; in the congregation I will praise you.

DAY 9 - RAISING YOUR AWARENESS

Romans 12:2-Do not be conformed to this world, but be transformed by the renewal of your mind, that by testing you may discern what is the will of God, what is good and acceptable and perfect.

2 Corinthians 4:16-So we do not lose heart. Though our outer self is wasting away, our inner self is being renewed day by day.

DAY 10 - COMING TO GRIPS WITH OUR SIN NATURE

1 Peter 5:8-Be sober-minded; be watchful. Your adversary the devil prowls around like a roaring lion, seeking someone to devour.

1 John 3:8-Whoever makes a practice of sinning is of the devil, for the devil has been sinning from the beginning. The reason the Son of God appeared was to destroy the works of the devil.

1 Corinthians 10:13-No temptation has overtaken you that is not common to man. God is faithful, and he will not let you be tempted beyond your ability, but with the temptation he will also provide the way of escape, that you may be able to endure it.

Romans 12:2-Do not be conformed to this world, but be transformed by the renewal of your mind, that by testing you may discern what is the will of God, what is good and acceptable and perfect.

DAY 11 - WHAT DO YOU BELIEVE?

1 John 4:1-Beloved, do not believe every spirit, but test the spirits to see whether they are from God, for many false prophets have gone out into the world.

Philippians 3:13-Brothers, I do not consider that I have made it my own. But one thing I do: forgetting what lies behind and straining forward to what lies ahead…

Romans 8:28-And we know that for those who love God all things work together for good, for those who are called according to his purpose.

DAY 12 AND 13 - TAKING RESPONSIBILITY

Matt 27:24-When Pilate saw that he was getting nowhere, but that instead an uproar was starting, he took water and washed his hands in front of the crowd. "I am innocent of this man's blood," he said. "It is your responsibility!"

Genesis 43:9-I myself will guarantee his safety; you can hold me personally responsible for him. If I do not bring him back to you and set him here before you, I will bear the blame before you all my life.

2 Sam 14:9-But the woman from Tekoa said to him, "My lord the king, let the blame rest on me and on my father's family, and let the king and his throne be without guilt."

DAY 14 - AVOIDING PROCRASTINATION

Psalm 34:4-I sought the LORD, and he answered me; he delivered me from all my fears.

Jos. 18:3-So Joshua said to the Israelites: "How long will you wait before you begin to take possession of the land that the Lord, the God of your fathers, has given you?"

2 Tim 1:7-For God did not give us a spirit of timidity, but a spirit of power, of love and of self-discipline.

DAY 15 - OVERCOMING EMOTIONAL EATING

Ephesians 6:12-For we do not wrestle against flesh and blood, but against the rulers, against the authorities, against the cosmic powers over this present darkness, against the spiritual forces of evil in the heavenly places.

Ephesians 4:26-Be angry and do not sin; do not let the sun go down on your anger

DAY 16 - SELF-IMAGE

Psalm 139:13-14-For you formed my inward parts; you knitted me together in my mother's womb. I praise you, for I am fearfully and wonderfully made.

Genesis 1:27-So God created man in his own image, in the image of God he created him; male and female he created them.

Ecclesiastes 3:11-He has made everything beautiful in its time. Also, he has put eternity into man's heart, yet so that he cannot find out what God has done from the beginning to the end.

Ephesians 2:10-For we are his workmanship, created in Christ Jesus for good works, which God prepared beforehand, that we should walk in them.

Genesis 1:31-And God saw everything that he had made, and behold, it was very good. And there was evening and there was morning, the sixth day.

DAY 17 - SELF- CONTROL

John 16:33-"I have told you these things, so that in me you may have peace. In this world you will have trouble. But take heart! I have overcome the world."

James 4:7-Submit yourselves, then, to God. Resist the devil, and he will flee from you

1 Peter 4:7-The end of all things is at hand; therefore be self-controlled and sober-minded for the sake of your prayers.

1 Corinthians 10:13-No temptation has overtaken you that is not common to man. God is faithful, and he will not let you be tempted beyond your ability, but with the temptation he will also provide the way of escape, that you may be able to endure it.

DAY 18 - STAYING FOCUSED

Psalm 119:15-I will meditate on your precepts and fix my eyes on your ways.

1 Corinthians 7:35-I say this for your own benefit, not to lay any restraint upon you, but to promote good order and to secure your undivided devotion to the Lord.

Philippians 4:8-Finally, brothers, whatever is true, whatever is honorable, whatever is just, whatever is pure, whatever is lovely, whatever is commendable, if there is any excellence, if there is anything worthy of praise, think about these things.

Proverbs 4:25-27-Let your eyes look straight ahead... Do not swerve to the right or the left

DAY 19 - PARTNERSHIPS

Ecclesiastes 4:9-12-Two are better than one, because they have a good reward for their toil. For if they fall, one will lift up his fellow. But woe to him who is alone when he falls and has not another to lift him up! Again, if two lie together, they keep warm, but how can one keep warm alone? And though a man might prevail against one who is alone, two will withstand him—a threefold cord is not quickly broken.

Proverbs 27:17-Iron sharpens iron, and one man sharpens another.

Matthew 18:20-For where two or three are gathered in my name, there am I among them.

DAY 20 -PRIORITIZING

Matthew 6:33-But seek first the kingdom of God and his righteousness, and all these things will be added to you.

Ecc. 10:2-The heart of the wise inclines to the right, but the heart of the fool to the left.

Matthew 6:21-For where your treasure is, there your heart will be also.

3 John 1:2-Beloved, I pray that all may go well with you and that you may be in good health, as it goes well with your soul.

DAY 21 - STAYING ON TRACK

James 2:18-But someone will say, "You have faith and I have works." Show me your faith apart from your works, and I will show you my faith by my works.

Proverbs 14:12-There is a way that seems right to a man, but its end is the way to death.

Psalm 119:105-Your word is a lamp to my feet and a light to my path.

ABOUT THE AUTHOR

Cathy Morenzie, a noted personal trainer, author, blogger and presenter, has been a leader in the faith/fitness industry for over half a decade. Her impact has influenced thousands of people over the years to help them lose weight and develop positive attitudes about their bodies and about fitness.

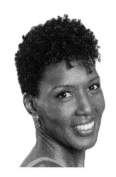

Over the years, she has seen some of the most powerful and faith-filled people struggle with their health and their weight. She wondered how it was possible for people to exercise so much power and authority, and yet feel so powerless in the area of health and fitness? How is it that we have been given the power and authority to cast out demons, yet we can't stop ourselves from eating a piece of chocolate? Why do we struggle with so many issues around our weight such as emotional eating, physical inactivity, self control, guilt and feelings and low-self esteem?

Cathy Morenzie herself - a rational, disciplined, faith-filled, personal trainer - struggled with her own weight, with emotional eating, self-doubt and low self-esteem. She tried to change just about everything about herself for much of her life so she knows what it's like to feel stuck.

Every insecurity, challenge and negative emotion that she experienced was equipping her to help other people who faced the same struggles - especially women.

With her Healthy by Design books and programs Cathy has helped thousands to learn to let go of their mental, emotional and spiritual bonds that have kept them stuck and instead rely on our heavenly father for true release from our fears, doubts, stress and anxieties. She also teaches people how to eat a sustainable healthy diet and find the motivation to exercise. Learn more at: www.cathymorenzie.com

Connect with Me

Friend me on Facebook:

www.facebook.com/cathymorenziechristianweightloss

Follow me on Twitter: **twitter.com/activeimage**

Subscribe to my blog: **www.cathymorenzie.com**

Join me in the *Weight Loss, God's Way Challenge*:

http://www.21daysgodsway.com

Book me to speak at your church, event or show

Every year I do a number of speaking engagements and media appearances. If you'd like me to come and speak at your church, event, webinar or on air about Christian weight loss principals and application you can learn more and contact me at:

www.cathymorenzie.com/contact-us

HEALTHY
by *Design*

21 DAY MEALPLAN

A Christian Women's
Guide to Stop Craving
Carbs and Lose Weight

Over 60 Delicious
Low-carb Recipes

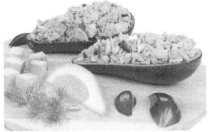
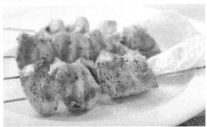
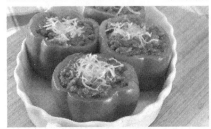
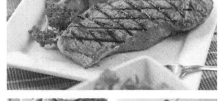
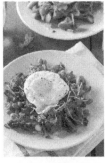
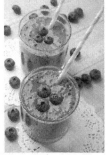

Cathy Morenzie

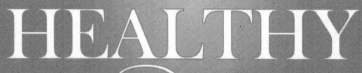

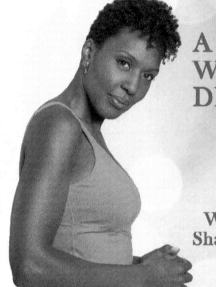

HEALTHY by Design

REFLECTIONS of GOD'S LOVE

A CHRISTIAN WEIGHT LOSS DEVOTIONAL

Includes
Weight Loss Prayers
Shares and Declarations

Cathy Morenzie

HEALTHY
by *Design*

TRAINER'S SECRETS

Real life success stories
show how to
lose weight,
get in shape,
and stay motivated
while strengthening
your faith in Christ.

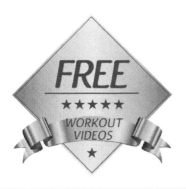

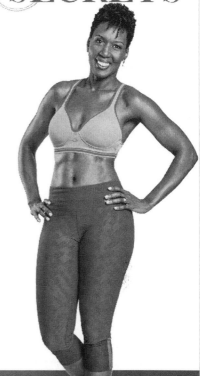

Cathy Morenzie

Made in the USA
Columbia, SC
07 September 2018